What Does Your Gut Tell You?

The Surefire Way to Get Rid of that Evil
Sagging Belly Fat

J.C. Collins

**Limits of Liability, Disclaimer of Warranties & Terms of
Use**
This book is a general educational health-related information
product. As an express condition to reading this book, you
understand and agree to following terms. The information and
advice contained in this book are not intended as a substitute for
consulting with a healthcare professional.

The publisher and authors are not responsible for any adverse
effects or consequences resulting from the use of any of the
suggestions, or procedures discussed in this book. While all
attempts have been made to verify information provided in this
book, the author and publisher assume no responsibility for
errors, omissions, or contrary interpretation of the subject
matter herein. All matters pertaining to your physical health
should be supervised by a health care professional

ISBN-10: 1500402222
ISBN-13: 978-1500402228

DEDICATION

This book is dedicated to those in search of an effective
way to get rid of that sagging belly fat…. for good.

CONTENTS

INTRODUCTION

Many of those in search of a way to lose weight fall into two categories - People who diet to lose weight and people who exercise to lose weight. Both are good ideas, but if you want to specifically target belly fat, you're going to have to do both.

Of course, the key to burning more calories throughout the day and revving up your metabolism is exercise. Putting that together with a healthy, low-calorie diet can give you more bang for your buck, helping you target that stubborn belly fat.

This book is dedicated to those in search of that very thing, an effective way to get rid of that sagging belly fat.... for good.

CHAPTER 1 – THE PATH TO EFFECTIVE BELLY FAT REDUCTION

We've all dreamed of having tight, toned stomachs with sexy six-packs, at some time in our lives. Abdominal weight is not only dangerous, it's just unfortunately, the hardest fat to get rid of. For many of us, tummy area seems to be the first place we attract extra pounds, and the last place that we are able to lose pounds.

While you may very well want to have a toned and flat belly, you may however, find it difficult to give up your favorite food items and to perform exercises on a regular basis.

Below are some of the most important guidelines on belly fat reduction that you need to keep in mind. By applying these guidelines in your regular routine, you will surely increase your chances of being successful in your efforts.

Avoid Carbonated Drinks

You have to eliminate drinking carbonated drinks as much as possible. This is not only limited to sodas. Aside from sodas, you should also stay away from energy drinks as much as possible. Diet sodas should also be restricted in your diet because they can also have detrimental effects on your current state of health.

Not only do these dehydrate your body and add calories without nutrition but also contribute in causing tummy bloating. As much as possible, you should also stay away from seltzer. As an alternative, you may try out drinking more plain water.

Stay Away from Salty Foods

Staying away from salty food items like chips and pretzels can help you avoid increasing belly fat. Chips and pretzels are just some of the most common food items that contain a lot of sodium. Sodium is considered as a substance that you can readily find in salt.

Because the aforementioned food items contain a lot of salt, your body will eventually retain extra fluid in the long run. Salt is considered as one of the contributing factors that can lead to weight gain. Aside from that, this substance can make you appear bloated not just in your belly but on other parts of your body.

Go for a Walk

You should take some time to talk to and walk with a friend. If you're going out for a walk, it's not a bad idea to have a companion to join you. Research shows that having an exercise buddy will encourage you to perform your simple exercises at a higher intensity, as compared to the exercise intensity that you have when you perform your routines alone.

You may plan a specific day and time when both of you are free for a gym session or a walking session. You may even end up organizing a fitness group in your neighborhood if you know a lot of people who are willing to participate in your cause. In this regard, you should recruit as many involved people as you can. In the process, you can highly encourage one another to do your best in your endeavors.

Fiber is Your Friend

If you want to see a decrease in belly fat levels, stay with food items that are rich in fiber. Amazingly, your belly can carry almost four percent less fat for every ten grams' worth of fiber that you can eat on a daily basis. Fortunately, there are a lot of easy ways that you can readily incorporate fiber in your diet. This is aside from eating a whole box of raisin bran.

The following are just some of the most common food items that contain at least ten grams of fiber that can help tighten your belly:

- Half a cup of pinto beans
- Two pieces of apples
- Two cups of broccoli
- Artichoke

Clean Your House (No, Really)

You can work out your abdominal muscles by doing simple chores around the house.

Cleaning the house may be considered as a hassle many people. However, while vacuuming your floor, you can incorporate different subtle workout routines in the activity as well.

When you vacuum, you can concentrate on contracting your abdomen while performing the drawing in maneuver. You can especially do this while you push the vacuum cleaner back and forth.

Avocado for Gut Busting

One of the most common belly fat busting food items that you can include in your diet regimen is the avocado.

Avocados are considered as one of the food items that are abundant in MUFAs (monosaturated fatty acids). Consuming just a half portion of an entire avocado can help you obtain around ten grams of this precious fatty acid. In the long run, this can help you prevent having spikes in your blood sugar levels. Therefore, you can suppress the tendency of your body to store all the fat on your abdominal region. To help you prevent the development of fat in your stomach, you should eat around ¼ cup of avocado per serving for your snacks or your meals.

Stay Active

You may focus on performing different sports activities to help you get rid of your belly fat.

Unknown to many, kayaking and canoeing can be considered as just some of the greatest abdominal workouts that you can definitely try out. For one thing, both of your upper and lower body region muscles can get intensive training because these are regarded as continuous activities with minimal rest periods. The muscles found on your abdomen and torso are constantly pulling, reaching, twisting, and stretching for prolonged periods of time.

Boxing is another sports activity that you may be interested to try out. You may try the conventional or aerobic kickboxing to help you tighten up your tummy muscles. These are not only good for your waistline measurement but also for your cardiovascular health. You just have to make sure that you will progress your exercise in case you already experience positive changes in your exercise regimen.

These are just some of the tips that you have to keep in mind if you want to get rid of your belly fat and keep it away for good. As impossible as it may seem, you can have a healthy and fit belly just by applying small changes in your daily routine. Let's continue…

J.C. Collins

CHAPTER 2 – THE IMPORTANCE OF EATING RIGHT

Eating the right types of food on a regular basis can help you lose a significant part of your belly fat. In the process, this can bring out the muscles that lie underneath that gut. Also, avoiding certain types of food items can help you get rid of the fat in no time.

This book section will discuss more about the food items that you need to consume and those that you have to avoid as much as possible. These are just some of the food items that you need to keep in mind. This is especially noteworthy for those items that you have to avoid on a long term basis.

Foods to Consume

Generally, the food items that you have to consume to get rid of the belly fat are those that encourage increased metabolism. While these food items allow your stomach to process the food more readily, this does not mean that the food items will be digested quickly. Ideal food items that can help you shed off those unwanted fats should encourage slow and consistent digestion and absorption. This way, you will not crave for inappropriate food items that will blow up your entire diet.

- *Black beans are legumes that are rich in fiber and protein.*

These are known as famous appetite reducers. Because of their dark color, the black beans are considered as one of the food items with really high flavonoid content among the beans. Studies show that these can help counteract the main mechanisms of your body that encourage the storage of excessive amounts of belly fat.

- *Cold potatoes are good alternatives to your well-loved potatoes if you do not feel like giving them up.*

For best results, you may even add some vinegar into the mix. If you chill these potatoes overnight, they will eventually form resistant starch crystals. These are fiber constituents that can help trigger the creation of hunger suppression hormones. Resistant starch can aid your body in getting rid of more belly fat that will eventually be used for fuel. At the same time, this can help create fewer amounts of fat that will be available for storage in different parts of your abdomen.

- *Pears are food items endowed with high levels of fiber and low amounts of calories.*

You may consume one of these before you have each of your meal and still keep on losing those unwanted pounds. These fruits are loaded with increased amounts of flavonoids and catechins. These are antioxidants that seem to hinder the belly fat storage. Studies have already proved this claim.

- *Interestingly, popcorn can be a good belly fat buster if you eat it without salt and butter.*

Additionally, the food item can help you lose a lot of belly fat because this belongs under the whole grain type. Research shows that people who consume higher amounts of whole grains eventually end up with midriffs of smaller girth than those who consume mostly refined varieties of grains.

Foods to Avoid

On the other hand, one of the most common characteristics of food items that you have to avoid is its ability to be broken down easily.

Food items with simple carbohydrates seem to be those that can your entire diet in jeopardy. These food items are easily processed and absorbed by the stomach and the small intestines before you know it. Because of this, you will go hungry more easily. In the long run, this can make you crave for more food items that you do not really need to eat at the moment. In the long run, this can just lead to build up of more belly fat.

- *Soda is not only a type of unhealthy beverage but one that can definitely increase the amount of fat in your belly.*

This contains empty calories that can increase your body weight further. Soda also contains insane amounts of sugars. These are derivatives of high fructose corn syrups and other types of additives. Unfortunately, your body typically has a hard time burning off this type of sugar. This especially applies to your midsection.

- *Pancakes can act as delicious breakfast treats but these contain large amounts of fats and calories.*

Consuming this type of food items can make you end up with more belly fat if you eat it with syrup. Even the light pancake varieties can lead to more belly fat in the long run. As much as possible, you need to avoid pancakes and learn to enjoy the whole wheat waffle instead. Studies have already shown that the whole wheat variety can lead to lower levels of belly fat.

- *While potato chips may be one of your most favorite food items, you need to ditch it if you want to end up with a slimmer tummy.*

Most of the brands of potato chips are cooked with hydrogenated oils. This is also known as a form of trans fat. Trans fat is well known because of its ability to increase the cholesterol levels inside your body. In the long run, this cannot only lead to increased body weight but also to higher risks of heart disease acquisition.

CHAPTER 3 – BENEFITS OF CARDIOVASCULAR EXERCISES

Many studies have shown that cardiovascular exercises can help you shed off great amounts of fat if you perform it consistently with the right intensity and frequency.

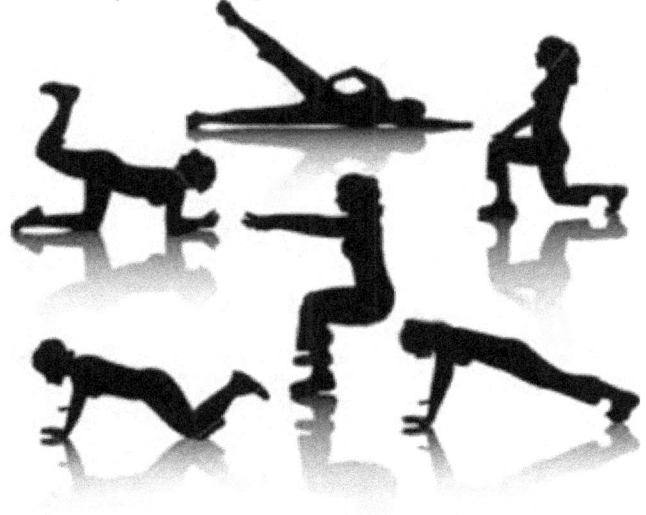

Here are some of the benefits of cardiovascular types of exercises to help you on your quest of belly fat destruction:

- **Cardiovascular exercises are also known as aerobic exercises.**

This type of exercise requires extensive oxygenated blood pumping by your heart. Eventually, the blood will be delivered to different muscles of your body. This includes the muscles in your trunk and abdomen.

Additionally, this can help stimulate your respiratory rate and heart rate because an increase in one of these components will definitely lead to the increase of the other vital sign. These are both sustained for the entire exercise duration.

These exercises do not only improve your overall fitness but also provide other benefits that can promote emotional and physical health. This includes the reduction of belly fat. Studies show that these exercises can help fight off the risks of having different types of cancers. On top of that, these can help prevent depression, diabetes, osteoporosis, and cardiovascular problems.

- **There are numerous physiological functions that get involved every time you perform these exercises.**

When you perform cardiovascular exercises, the entire process starts off with breathing. The breathing pattern takes on a normal rate. This means that your body takes in and gets rid of air of around 7 to 8 liters in a minute.

Your heart will also pump blood at a faster rate as well. Every heartbeat sends off a certain blood volume along with other life sustaining nutrients like oxygen. This is required because your muscles will need more of these nutrients due to an increased need for energy.

Because of a faster exchange of nutrients taken in and waste materials taken out of your system, your digestive system will have a faster metabolic rate. In the long run, this will make it easier for your body systems to get rid of the stored fat located in different parts of your body. This includes your belly fat.

- **Like other types of exercises, aerobic exercises have routines that you have to follow.**

This is important because if you perform aerobic exercises with excessively high intensity, you will end up having muscle cramps and other similar types of injuries in the future. These arise because of unwarranted fatigue.

For starters, you have to continuously perform your aerobic exercises for at least 20 minutes. Because 20 minutes is relatively long, you have to consider significantly lowering the intensity of the exercise routine that you have to perform. This is also the reason that you have to stay away from free weights and other forms of resistance for these exercises.

As for advanced exercise enthusiasts, this initial routine is slightly increased. Experts recommend you to perform these exercises for three to five times in a week. Within six to eight weeks, you will start seeing the effects of these exercises on your belly fat.

- **Cardiovascular exercises are useless if you cannot progress them to a certain level.**

Progressing in this type of exercise is pretty easy. Initially, you have to determine the baseline measurement of your exercise routine. If you obtained 20 minutes as your baseline, you may add five more minutes to your aerobic exercises sessions in a week.

In case you have already seen some improvements on your exercises in terms of overall endurance, you may want to add in five more minutes to the total exercise time. You may do this until you have reached 45 minutes' worth of continuous exercise time in a session.

The entire concept of progression may sound too easy. However, you should keep in mind that the changes that you will experience because of these exercises will only be initially dramatic. Therefore, you should not feel discouraged if aerobic exercise progression is still not warranted on your part.

There are different types of aerobic exercises that you may be interested to try out.

To help you stay motivated in getting rid of your belly fat, you have to choose the type of cardiovascular exercise that closely fits in with your interest. According to experts, if you want to get rid of belly fat through these exercises, you have to go for moderate intensity. This is also your plan of action if you are in the maintenance phase.

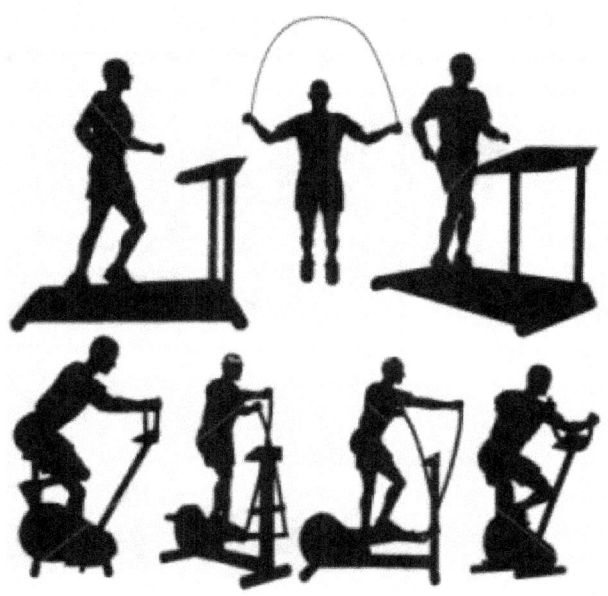

- Running is considered as an inexpensive form of aerobic exercise.

- If you want to get rid of belly fat but do not want to get exposed to the heat, you may want to go for swimming.

- In case you want an activity that seems more intensive than swimming, you may go for aquarobics.

- Cycling is another workout that you may try, especially if you are suffering from knee problems.

- Rowing is a low impact alternative to cycling or running that can help you target numerous parts of your body, including your belly.

- Boxing can not only help you get rid of belly fat but can also help develop your upper body strength.

These are just some of the most common concepts that you need to know and learn about cardiovascular exercises. I would highly encourage you to include this in the roster of exercise routines that you are planning to perform soon because this can help you improve the success rate of the entire program.

CHAPTER 4- BENEFITS OF
RESISTANCE EXERCISES

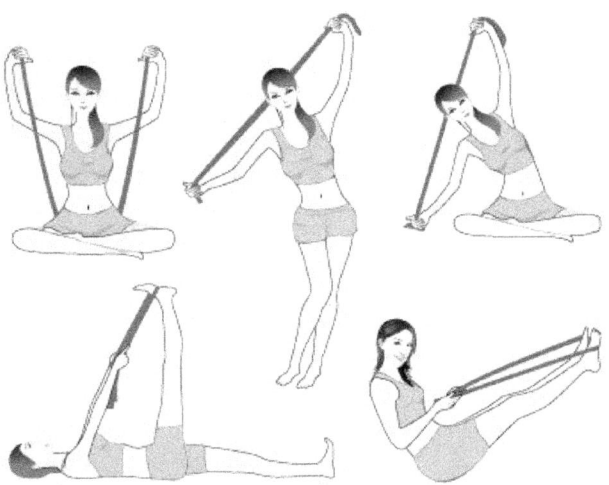

Strengthening or resistance exercises for your abdominal region can be just as effective in helping your reduce belly fat. This is in comparison with the cardiovascular exercises. Here are some of the most important types of strengthening exercises that can help you achieve positive results within four to six weeks.

1- Drawing-in Maneuver

The drawing in maneuver can help you significantly strengthen your core muscle group.

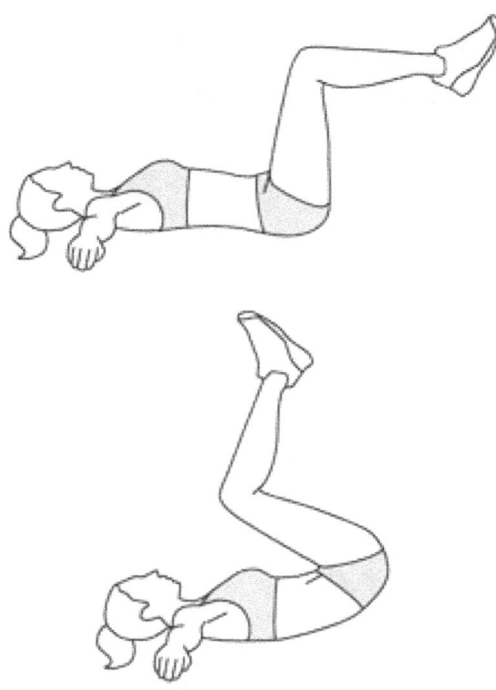

- The drawing in maneuver targets the quadrates lumborum. This is also known as the corset muscle group. To perform this exercise, you have to assume the hook lying position. After this, you have to move your belly button upward and inward. However, you have to perform this gradually so as to minimize the activation of other adjacent abdominal muscle groups.

- You have to perform the hold for approximately five to ten seconds with five repetitions per set. You are encouraged to perform this exercise at the beginning of each exercise session to help you maximize the belly fat busting effects of the other exercises that you have included in your program.

  Still, you are encouraged to perform this activity even if you are doing other tasks or other exercise routines. In the long run, this can help you improve the stability of your trunk while getting rid of your belly fat.

2- Planks

- Planks are deceptively difficult exercises that can help you improve your abdominal muscle strength while giving your midriff some muscle definition.

- If you will view some of the images related to this exercise, you may have an impression that this is an easy routine for you. Well, that is until you try it for yourself. Planks are all about stability. Therefore, a specific part of your body should work really hard to keep your body in equilibrium to maintain a certain position. In this case, your belly muscles are tasked to work double time.

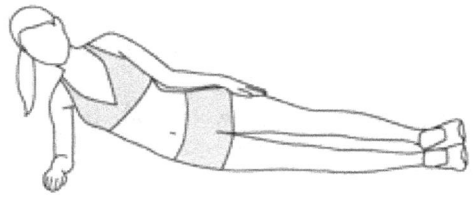

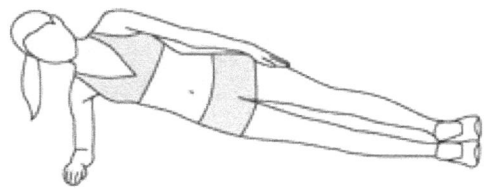

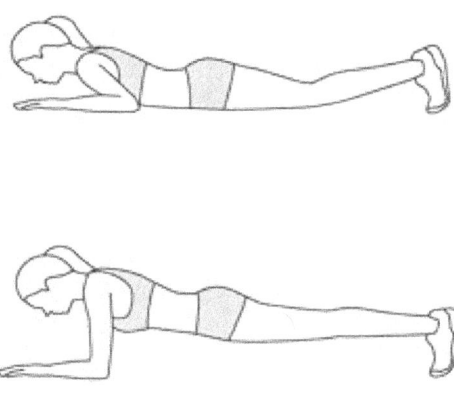

- To perform this exercise, you need to assume the push up position. However, instead of having both of your arms outstretched, you need to keep your elbows bent at around 90 degrees. Also, you should make sure that your forearms are in contact with the exercise surface. You should hold the position for 10 seconds. You may progress this exercise until you can manage to hold the position for one minute per repetition.

3- Sit Ups

Sit up is one of the most common but one of the most difficult strengthening exercises that you may perform to target your belly fat.

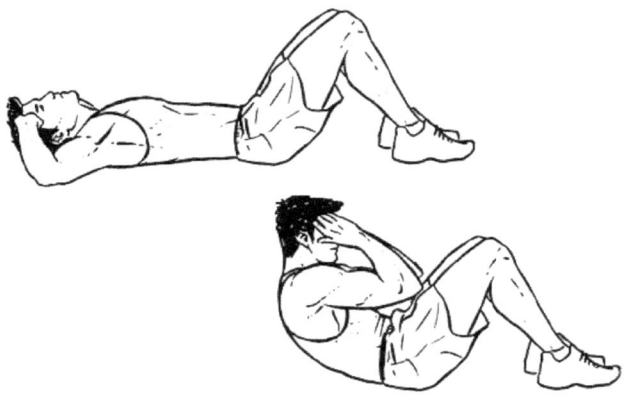

- Like the drawing in maneuver, you should start off this routine in hook lying position. While most of the traditional workout buffs may encourage you to lift your trunk as far as you can, you should only aim to clear your shoulder blades off the exercises surface. Going beyond this point will only activate the adjacent muscle groups otherthan your belly muscles.

- There are three forms of progression for the exercise. These are determined according to your arm positioning while performing the exercise. If you are a beginner, you should cross your arms over your chest. If you think you can already take the exercise to another level, you should make sure that you will cup your hands at the back of your neck while your arms are fully bent. For advanced exercise enthusiasts, you have to stretch your arms overhead. You may further progress the exercise by holding free weights on both hands while stretching your arms overhead.

4- Diagonal Sit Ups

Diagonal sit ups are considered as modifications of the previous exercise.

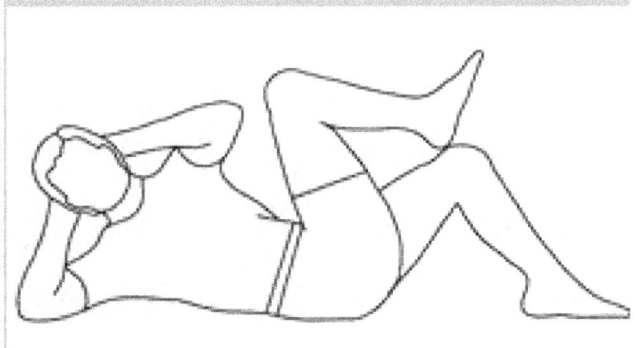

- If the sit ups mainly focus on your rectus abdominis to help you get rid of your belly fat, the diagonal counterpart work on the lateral muscles of your belly to help in significantly removing the fat. The same exercise dosimetry applies for this exercise as well.

- To perform this exercise, you also have to start off by positioning yourself in hook lying position. If you are planning to work out the right part of your trunk, you should lift your right shoulder in an attempt to reach for your left knee. After this, you should go for the left muscle group of your belly by performing the opposite movement. You should perform a minimum of ten repetitions and two sets for this type of exercise routine. For beginners, rest periods of ten seconds in between sets are recommended.

5- Leg Raises

If you are too lazy to lift your trunk to execute belly exercises, you may give the leg raises a shot.

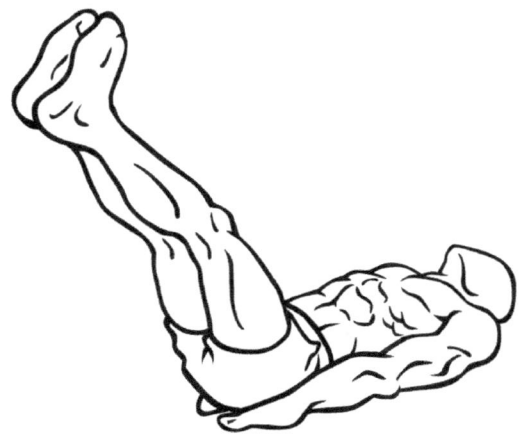

- Leg raises are exercise routines that can help make your abdominal muscles work without creating too much of a tension for the rest of your adjacent muscles. This can work especially well for the lower abdominal region. The extent that this will work for this region will highly depend on the angle where you will hold both of your feet in raised position. A higher lower extremity to trunk angle will cause more work to take place on lower muscle groups of your belly.

- First, you should position yourself in supine position. Your hands should be positioned at the small of your back. You have to make sure that you are lying down on a stable surface. For one repetition, you need to stretch out both of your legs and lift them such that they create a 90 degree angle with your trunk. You have to perform the leg raising movement as fast as you can.

  Then bring down both of your feet after the repetition, you should gradually do this. Slowly bringing down your feet after every repetition will help you maximize the eccentric muscle contraction for your abdomen. This means that your trunk muscle groups will be strengthened even more.

CHAPTER 5 – NATURAL REMEDIES TO REDUCE BELLY FAT

While overall weight loss is the only known way to fight abdominal obesity and protect against obesity-related diseases, some research suggests that certain natural solutions may help reduce belly fat. Here's a look at several study findings:

Almonds

One of the best ways to naturally lose belly fat is the inclusion of almonds in your diet; it can be of great help. It also helps your body in the protection against diabetes, cardiovascular diseases, cancer and more importantly weight gain and obesity.

Almonds are also a great source of protein and fiber. In other to lose weight and to get a flat belly, sprinkle 2 tablespoons of almonds over an unsweetened yogurt and berries. This can be taken as a morning meal.

Garlic

In order to reduce belly fat, chew 3-4 cloves of raw garlic in the morning and drink the lemon water after consuming garlic. This is one of the best home remedies to reduce belly fat.

Eggs

Egg is loaded with plenty of vitamins and contains calcium, zinc, iron, phosphorus, omega-3, etc. All these vitamins are credited to helping reduce belly fat. So, grab an omelette in the morning for a flat belly.

Yoghurt

Apart from the fact that it is low in calories and fat, it also helps to aid digestion. It promotes the growth of bacteria in the gut and help to combat excess gas and bloating. It is very low in fat, for this reason, it fits into any diet plan either as part of a meal or even a snack between meals. I recommend you to combine it with flax seeds as a morning smoothie.

Fruits and Vegetables

- **Apple**

Eating apple regularly can help in fighting many diseases and it can also help in reducing the fat from your belly. Apple helps your stomach to feel full because it contains potassium and many vitamins. So, eat an apple in breakfast to get the desired tummy size.

- **Watermelon**

Watermelon contains 82% water, which helps your stomach not to crave for food. Watermelon is rich in vitamin C, which is beneficial for health.

- **Bananas**

Like apples, bananas are also rich in potassium and contain multivitamins. They are filling and help you to resist the cravings for fast food. Moreover, banana boosts the metabolic rate, thereby melting the belly fat.

- **Avocados**

This is a great source of Mono Unsaturated Fatty Acids (MUFAs), just like flax seeds, it contains more of beta-sitosterol - the cholesterol smashing chemical - than any other fruits, thereby lowering the cholesterol level in the body. Beta sitosterol has also been found to ease symptoms of benign prostatic enlargement and the prevention of oxidative damage through its antioxidant activity. Add about a quarter cup of mashed avocado with lime juice, salt and pepper and serve with raw vegetables to get the best out of this belly flattening fruit.

- **Beans and Legumes**

Jam packed full of natural protein and soluble fiber, beans and legumes are the perfect replacement for meat protein as you cut out the unsaturated fats and in turn replenish your body with fibers that gel with water keeping your appetite at bay and energy levels nice and consistent.

- **Celery**

Celery also helps in reducing the fat from the belly and it contains only 8 calories. Drink celery juice or eat raw celery as a salad.

The Wonders of Natural Herbs

Numerous problems in the human body can be addressed with the help of herbs and their supplements. There are also a few herbs that help shed the extra pounds and maintain ideal weight. Here are some herbs that help reduce the pudginess around the belly.

- *Cayenne*

  Cayenne is a rich source of capsaicin that belongs to the family of hot chili peppers. This chemical compound helps generate body heat, which initiates the faster burning of fat. It also acts as an appetite suppressant, thereby reducing the feeling of hunger.

- *Chickweed*

  Used as a herbal remedy to melt the extra fat around the belly and thighs. Chickweed can be taken in the form of decoction, this herb effectively burns fat and releases energy. Other illnesses that can be relieved with the use of chickweed are rheumatic pains, constipation, wounds and ulcers etc.

- *Dandelion*

  Prescribed to people who are keen on shedding off the extra pounds around the waist. The leaves and flowers of the dandelion plant are used as a herbal remedy. Loaded with vitamins and calcium, this herb acts as a diuretic and laxative as well. Dandelion controls the craving for sweets, which are a cause for belly fat.

- *Ginger*

    Ginger root is also a popular herb that triggers the burning of extra calories which in turn helps reduce belly fat. Since more energy is used by the tissues for calorie burning, the level of cholesterol is controlled. Ginger also helps improve the functioning of the joints and in several other health conditions.

- *Ginseng*

    Popular as a metabolism booster, ginseng also helps increase energy levels in the body. It also increases the endurance of the body against a number of ailments, people who have a tendency to retain excess water in the body or who are overweight are recommended to take ginseng, for a healthy weight loss.

Green Tea Extract

Drinking a cup of green tea twice a day is known to reduce belly fat and also keep it trimmed down. It helps boost the rate of metabolism thereby increase the burning of calories in the body. Not only this, green tea is also considered to be an excellent source of antioxidants, which helps the body fight against the free radicals thus preventing infections and diseases, and also keep them at bay.

CHAPTER 6 – ADAPTING TO LIFESTYLE CHANGES

Even if you have the perfect diet program and the flawless exercise regimen, you cannot get rid of your belly fat if you keep on applying the same type of lifestyle that you have always been used to. In this book section, you will learn more about the lifestyle changes that you have to implement in your life so you can finally get rid of your belly fat.

Stay Hydrated

- *Hydration is important no matter what type of diet and exercise regimen you are participating in at the moment.*

- Staying hydrated is considered crucial in maintaining the normal functions of your body. However, studies show that drinking down lots of water can aid in shedding off the pounds at a faster rate. This is usually because water can help you stay full for longer periods. Because of this, you will consume less food within a given period of time.

- As much as possible, you should try to drink eight glasses of water in a day at the very least. Furthermore, you drink one to two glasses of water before your meals. This will help you feel fuller at a faster rate. You can also suppress your appetite because of this.

Don't Skip a Meal

- *As much as possible, you should avoid skipping meals.*

- While it may appear counterintuitive, not skipping your meals can help you lose a significant amount of stored belly fat by slowing down your metabolic rate. One of the best methods to speed up your metabolic rate is to consume small portions of food with regular meal intervals. In other words, you are better off eating six small meals in a day rather than eating two or three large ones.

Monitor Your Progress

- *Constant monitoring is important so you can see if your regimen is working to help you get rid of your belly fat.*

- Initially, you can do this by taking down the baseline measurements of your waist line. You should do this before you start off with your diet and exercise program so you can have a certain value where you can compare your current measurements.

- To obtain the required values for baseline, you need to measure first around your lower belly then the narrowest part of the waist. Your lower belly measurement should be taken around one inch beneath the belly button.

- You need to weigh yourself at least once a week to help you keep track of your progress. For accurate results, you should take your measurements in the morning before you eat or drink anything. As much as possible, you should also take the measurements without clothes or in your underwear.

Get a Workout Buddy

- *If you are having a hard time getting started with your exercise program, you may seek help from someone you truly trust.*

- Shedding off the unwanted pounds in your own may be difficult when the people around you are usually consuming unhealthy food items. This becomes even harder if they pressure you to join them. Finding a friend whom you can exercise with or diet with can help you stay motivated during your endeavor. You may even share your tricks and tips with this person and ask one another to continue with the regimen.

- This lifestyle change can work even better if you see yourself as a competitive person. To further improve the effect of this change, you may even place some bets with your friends to see who will get rid of the belly fat at a faster rate.

Start a Journal

- *A diet journal can help you monitor your progress further.*

- Studies show that those who usually keep track of the food item that they eat by listing down the food items tend to shed off the unwanted belly fats at a faster rate. They also tend to keep this weight off than those who do not do anything to monitor the food items that they take in. This slightly because of the fact that writing down the food items makes you accountable for most of your food choice decisions.

- If you want to be objective about monitoring your food items, you should use the online calorie diary or calculator like Calorie King or My Fitness Pal. These sites can most likely help you monitor the food items that you eat on a regular basis. Also, this can permit you to check out the caloric content of different food items that you plan to consume in the future.

Sleep Some More

- *Believe it or not, having more sleep can help you get rid of your belly fat.*

- In case you are interested to work during the wee hours of the night, you should think again. When your biorhythms tare turned off, you will end up consuming more than what you are used to. When you lack sleep and you feel tired, your body will produce heightened levels of ghrelin. Ghrelin acts as a trigger that will enhance your craving for fat building food items such as sugar.

- On the other hand, losing a lot of sleep can contribute to alteration of hormone production. In turn, this can lead to the affectation of cortisol levels that will eventually lead to the insulin sensitivity of your body. In the long run, this can greatly contribute to the development of belly fat. This is one of the reasons that having at least seven hours of sleep per night is considered as one of the greatest things that you can change in your lifestyle so you can get rid of a significant level of belly fat.

The Importance of Stress Management

Managing your stress is one of the major lifestyle changes that you can do to significantly reduce the amount of fat that you have in your belly.

You need to quit telling yourself off and determine what you need to be happy. By recognizing how you can manage your stress, you are also paving a way to get rid of your belly fat for good. This is particularly important to implement in your workplace.

You are trying to gain control over the stress levels of your body, then you have to get the fundamentals right.

If you think about it, exercise, hydration, sleep, and good nutrition can help you lay out the foundation for your body and mind to cope up with numerous stressful situations. You will eventually realize that as you feel stronger because of better stress coping mechanisms, the original concerns that cause your stress is not as overpowering or vivid as you have thought of it before.

Writing down your plan on how you can manage your stress levels may feel like adding up another item on your to do list.

However, you should keep in mind that this can serve as your guide to frequently check yourself against. You should work on what will help you feel better. If you think that your strategy will work on your case to get rid of your belly fat, you should plan to incorporate this in your daily life by all means. If you think that you will feel calmer on the days that you have spent a significant amount of tie outside, then you should include an additional 30 minute walk to your schedule. Moreover, you need to stick to this initial plan.

To help you make the stress management plan more effective for you in the work place, you need to make sure that you will plan out your strategies with your manager.

This is important because this can help both parties determine the expectations that they need to have from each other. In the process, this can help them in significantly reducing the anxiety levels for both sides. Composing a written plan can also help you review and monitor the actions and approach that you have committed to do.

These are just some of the lifestyle changes that you have to apply in your life. In case you are not sure if a certain lifestyle change is applicable for you, you need to consult your physician about this. This is especially important if you think you are suffering from any form of chronic diseases such as hypertension and heart attack.

A FINAL WORD

So, how do you get rid of that sagging belly fat? Well... not by investing tons of money into fancy gadgets, expensive pills, and starving oneself, but it's in nourishing the body, eliminating the impurities and exercising. You won't have a model-ready body by tomorrow, but in time you will lose the belly fat and keep it off.

Don't try to change your lifestyle overnight by doing too much, too fast. Start by making small changes like drinking more water, eating more fresh fruits and vegetables, and going for a walk a few days a week. Once you get used to it, you'll start to feel better and you'll want to do more of these things because you'll be seeing results.

Small changes, if you do them often, can build up like a snowball and create huge changes in the future.

Please Leave a Review

Finally, if you enjoyed this book, please take the time to share your thoughts and post a review on Amazon. It would be greatly appreciated.

That review and feedback will help me improve the content in my books – and make each and every one more relevant and helpful to you.

Thank you again and good luck!

J.C. Collins